Contents

What is cholesterol?

Cholesterol is a type of lipid. It's a waxy, fat-like substance that your liver produces naturally. It's vital for the formation of cell membranes, certain hormones, and vitamin D.

Cholesterol doesn't dissolve in water, so it can't travel through your blood on its own. To help transport cholesterol, your liver produces lipoproteins.

Lipoproteins are particles made from fat and protein. They carry cholesterol and triglycerides (another type of lipid) through your bloodstream. The two major forms of lipoprotein are low-density lipoprotein (LDL) and high-density lipoprotein (HDL).

If your blood contains too much LDL cholesterol (cholesterol carried by low-density lipoprotein), it's known as high cholesterol. When left untreated, high cholesterol can lead to many health problems, including heart attack or stroke.

High cholesterol typically causes no symptoms. That's why it's important to get your cholesterol levels checked on a regular basis.

LDL cholesterol, or "bad cholesterol"

Low-density lipoprotein (LDL) is often called "bad cholesterol." It carries cholesterol to your arteries. If your levels of LDL cholesterol are too high, it can build up on the walls of your arteries.

The buildup is also known as cholesterol plaque. This plaque can narrow your arteries, limit your blood flow, and raise your risk of blood clots. If a blood clot blocks an artery in your heart or brain, it can cause a heart attack or stroke.

According to the Centers for Disease Control and PreventionTrusted Source, over one-third of American adults have elevated levels of LDL cholesterol.

HDL cholesterol, or "good cholesterol"

High-density lipoprotein (HDL) is sometimes called "good cholesterol." It helps return LDL cholesterol to your liver to be removed from your body. This helps prevent cholesterol plaque from building up in your arteries.

When you have healthy levels of HDL cholesterol, it can help lower your risk of blood clots, heart disease, and stroke.

Triglycerides, a different type of lipid

Triglycerides are another type of lipid. They're different from cholesterol. While your body uses cholesterol to build cells and certain hormones, it uses triglycerides as a source of energy.

When you eat more calories than your body can use right away, it converts those calories into triglycerides. It stores triglycerides in your fat cells. It also uses lipoproteins to circulate triglycerides through your bloodstream.

If you regularly eat more calories than your body can use, your triglyceride levels can get high.

This may raise your risk of several health problems, including heart disease and stroke.

Your doctor can use a simple blood test to measure your triglyceride level, as well as your cholesterol levels.

Getting your cholesterol levels checked

If you're age 20 years or older, the American Heart Association recommends getting your cholesterol levels checked at least once every four to six years. If you have a history of high cholesterol or other risk factors for cardiovascular disease, your doctor may encourage you get your cholesterol levels tested more often.

Your doctor can use a lipid panel to measure your total cholesterol level, as well your LDL cholesterol, HDL cholesterol, and triglyceride levels. Your total cholesterol level is the overall amount of cholesterol in your blood. It includes LDL and HDL cholesterol.

If your levels of total cholesterol or LDL cholesterol are too high, your doctor will diagnose you with high cholesterol. High cholesterol is especially dangerous when your LDL levels are too high and your HDL levels are too low.

Recent guidelines for normal cholesterol levels

Your body needs some cholesterol to function properly, including some LDL. But if your LDL levels are too high, it can raise your risk of serious health problems.

In 2013, the American College of Cardiologists (ACC) and the American Heart Association (AHA) developed new guidelines for the treatment of high cholesterol.

Before this change, doctors would manage cholesterol based on numbers in a cholesterol levels chart. Your doctor would measure your total cholesterol, HDL cholesterol, and LDL cholesterol levels. They would then decide whether to prescribe a cholesterol-lowering medication based on how your numbers compared to the numbers in the chart.

Under the new guidelines, in addition to your cholesterol levels, treatment recommendations consider other risk factors for heart disease. These risk factors include diabetes and the estimated 10-year risk for a cardiac event such as a heart attack or stroke. So what your "normal" cholesterol levels are depends on whether you have other risk factors for heart disease.

These new guidelines recommend that if you don't have risk factors for heart disease, your doctor should prescribe treatment if your LDL is greater than 189 mg/dL. To find out what your personal cholesterol recommendations are, talk to your doctor.

Cholesterol levels chart

With the changes mentioned above in the treatment guidelines for high cholesterol,

cholesterol charts are no longer considered the best way for doctors to gauge the management of cholesterol levels in adults.

However, for the average child and adolescent, the National Heart, Lung, and Blood InstituteTrusted Source classifies cholesterol levels (mg/dL) as follows:

High cholesterol symptoms

In most cases, high cholesterol is a "silent" problem. It typically doesn't cause any symptoms. Many people don't even realize they have high cholesterol until they develop serious complications, such as a heart attack or stroke.

That's why routine cholesterol screening is important. If you're age 20 years or older, ask your doctor if you should have routine cholesterol screening.

Causes of high cholesterol

Eating too many foods that are high in cholesterol, saturated fats, and trans fats may increase your risk of developing high cholesterol. Other lifestyle factors can also contribute to high cholesterol. These factors include inactivity and smoking.

Your genetics can also affect your chances of developing high cholesterol. Genes are passed down from parents to children. Certain genes instruct your body on how to process cholesterol and fats. If your parents have high cholesterol, you're at higher risk of having it too.

In rare cases, high cholesterol is caused by familial hypercholesterolemia. This genetic disorder prevents your body from removing LDL. According to the National Human Genome Research Institute, most adults with this condition have total cholesterol levels above 300 mg/dL and LDL levels above 200 mg/dL.

Other health conditions, such as diabetes and hypothyroidism, may also increase your risk of developing high cholesterol and related complications.

Risk factors for high cholesterol

You may be at a higher risk of developing high cholesterol if you:

- are overweight or obese

- eat an unhealthy diet

- don't exercise regularly

- smoke tobacco products

- have a family history of high cholesterol

- have diabetes, kidney disease, or hypothyroidism

People of all ages, genders, and ethnicities can have high cholesterol.

Complications of high cholesterol

If left untreated, high cholesterol can cause plaque to build up in your arteries. Over time, this plaque can narrow your arteries. This condition is known as atherosclerosis.

Atherosclerosis is a serious condition. It can limit the flow of blood through your arteries. It also raises your risk of developing dangerous blood clots.

Atherosclerosis can result in many life-threatening complications, such as:

- stroke

- heart attack

- angina (chest pain)

- high blood pressure

- peripheral vascular disease

- chronic kidney disease

High cholesterol can also create a bile imbalance, raising your risk of gallstones.

How to diagnose high cholesterol

To measure your cholesterol levels, your doctor will use a simple blood test. It's known as a lipid panel. They can use it to assess your levels of total cholesterol, LDL cholesterol, HDL cholesterol, and triglycerides.

To conduct this test, your doctor or other healthcare professional will take a sample of your blood. They will send this sample to a lab for analysis. When your test results become available, they will let you know if your cholesterol or triglyceride levels are too high.

To prepare for this test, your doctor may ask you to avoid eating or drinking anything for at least 12 hours beforehand.

How to lower cholesterol

If you have high cholesterol, your doctor may recommend lifestyle changes to help lower it. For instance, they may recommend changes to your diet, exercise habits, or other aspects of your daily routine. If you smoke tobacco products, they will likely advise you to quit.

Your doctor may also prescribe medications or other treatments to help lower your cholesterol levels. In some cases, they may refer you to a specialist for more care.

Lowering cholesterol through diet

To help you achieve and maintain healthy cholesterol levels, your doctor may recommend changes to your diet.

For example, they may advise you to:

• limit your intake of foods that are high in cholesterol, saturated fats, and trans fats

• choose lean sources of protein, such as chicken, fish, and legumes

• eat a wide variety of high-fiber foods, such as fruits, vegetables, and whole grains

• opt for baked, broiled, steamed, grilled, and roasted foods instead of fried foods

• avoid fast food and junk food

Foods that are high in cholesterol, saturated fats, or trans fats include:

• red meat, organ meats, egg yolks, and high-fat dairy products

• processed foods made with cocoa butter, palm oil, or coconut oil

• deep fried foods, such as potato chips, onion rings, and fried chicken

• certain baked goods, such as some cookies and muffins

Eating fish and other foods that contain omega-3 fatty acids may also help lower your LDL levels. For example, salmon, mackerel, and herring are rich sources of omega-3s. Walnuts, almonds, ground flax seeds, and avocados also contain omega-3s.

Cholesterol medications

In some cases, your doctor might prescribe medications to help lower your cholesterol levels.

Statins are the most commonly prescribed medications for high cholesterol. They block your liver from producing more cholesterol.

Examples of statins include:

- atorvastatin (Lipitor)

- fluvastatin (Lescol)

- rosuvastatin (Crestor)

- simvastatin (Zocor)

Your doctor may also prescribe other medications for high cholesterol, such as:

- niacin

- bile acid resins or sequesterants, such as colesevalam (Welchol), colestipol (Colestid), or cholestyramine (Prevalite)

- cholesterol absorption inhibitors, such as ezetimibe (Zetia)

Some products contain a combination of drugs to help decrease your body's absorption of cholesterol from foods and reduce your liver's production of cholesterol. One example is a combination of ezetimibe and simvastatin (Vytorin). Learn more about the drugs used to treat high cholesterol.

How to lower cholesterol naturally

In some cases, you may be able to lower your cholesterol levels without taking medications. For example, it may be enough to eat a nutritious diet, exercise regularly, and avoid smoking tobacco products.

Some people also claim that certain herbal and nutritional supplements may help lower cholesterol levels. For instance, such claims have been made about:

- garlic

- hawthorn

- astragalus

- red yeast rice

- plant sterol and stanol supplements

- oat bran, found in oatmeal and whole oats

- blond psyllium, found in psyllium seed husk

- ground flax seed

However, the level of evidence supporting these claims varies. Also, the U.S. Food and Drug Administration (FDA) hasn't approved any of these products for treating high cholesterol. More research is needed to learn if they can help treat this condition.

Always talk to your doctor before taking any herbal or nutritional supplements. In some cases, they might interact with other medications you're taking.

How to prevent high cholesterol

Genetic risk factors for high cholesterol can't be controlled. However, lifestyle factors can be managed.

To lower your risk of developing high cholesterol:

- Eat a nutritious diet that's low in cholesterol and animal fats, and high in fiber.

- Avoid excessive alcohol consumption.

- Maintain a healthy weight.

- Exercise regularly.

- Don't smoke.

You should also follow your doctor's recommendations for routine cholesterol screening. If you're at risk of high cholesterol or coronary heart disease, they will likely encourage you to get your cholesterol levels tested on a regular basis.

How It Works

When you're thinking about how much cholesterol is in your diet, remember that your body makes its own supply—and it will provide what you need, despite your diet. As such, there isn't a set amount of cholesterol you need to get from the food you eat.

In the past, the general recommendation was 300 milligrams (mg) of dietary cholesterol (or less) per day. However, in 2018, the American Heart Association guidelines for dietary cholesterol intake were changed.

Most adults, whether they have high cholesterol or not, are advised to keep dietary cholesterol intake low while still eating a varied, balanced, and "heart-healthy" diet, but adherence to these guidelines is especially important if you've been prescribed a diet for high cholesterol.

Your doctor may make more specific recommendations for you based on your overall health (for example, if you have other chronic health conditions or risk factors for heart disease).

Duration

Once you've made changes to the way you eat to help manage your cholesterol, you'll likely need to keep those changes long term; going back to your previous diet may encourage your levels to rise again.

Given this, it may help to think about your new way of eating as a permanent lifestyle modification rather than a temporary diet.

What to Eat

Focus on foods high in soluble fiber, phytosterols, and protein. Swap foods high in saturated or trans fats for those with unsaturated fats.

Compliant Foods

- Spinach, lettuce, kale

- Kiwi

- Oranges

- Grapefruit

- Apples

- Pears

- Plums

- Grapes

- Carrots

- Beets

- Rutabaga

- Cucumbers

- Celery

- Peppers

- Avocados

- High-fiber whole grains

- Margarine

- Barley

- Oatmeal

- Bulgar

- Quinoa

- Lentils

- Brown rice

- Turkey

- Tofu

- Chicken

- Halibut

- Cod

- Tilapia

- Tuna

- Salmon

- Egg whites or egg substitutes

- Almonds, walnuts

- Sesame and pumpkin seeds

- Sterol/stanol-fortified foods

Non-Compliant Foods

- Beef

- Liver

- Sausage

- Bacon

- Bologna

- Duck

- Goose

- Beef jerky

- Salami

- Canned fish packed in oil

- Hot dogs

- Shellfish

- Shrimp

- Pork

- Egg yolks

- Gravy

- Milk

- Cheese

- Whole milk yogurt

- Doughnuts, pastries, cookies, cakes

- Packaged snack food

- Ice cream

- Pudding

- Creamy sauces

- Soft drinks

- Fruit juice with sugar

- Fried food/fast food

- Coconut oil, palm kernel oil

- Butter, lard, shortening

- Partially hydrogenated or hydrogenated vegetable oil

- Buttered popcorn, potato chips, pretzels

- Alcohol (mixed drinks, cocktails)

Fruits and vegetables: Plants don't contain any dietary cholesterol, so you won't have to limit fruits and vegetables in your diet. Aside from being nutritious, fruits and veggies are also packed with fiber and phytosterols—healthy chemicals that help you to keep your LDL levels in check.

Salads are typical go-tos, but be mindful of what you top them with. To give a salad lipid-lowering power, skip the dressing and extras like bacon, and go for a mix of leafy greens, lean protein, and seeds.

Grains: Soluble fiber can reduce the amount of cholesterol you absorb and lower LDL. Whole-grain foods (breads, flours, rice) are typically higher in fiber than their refined counterparts; oats and oat bran are particularly great choices.

However, check food labels for the fiber content and total carbohydrate content, since some already-prepared grains may contain added sugars.

Protein: You can eat meat on a lipid-lowering diet, just be careful about the types that you include. While the recommendations have long been to avoid red meat and choose lean white meat instead, a 2019 study published in the American Journal of Clinical Nutrition found that red meat and white meat didn't differ much in terms of how they affected cholesterol levels.

Fish such as halibut, tilapia, and cod are low in fat and carbohydrates and high in protein. Tuna and salmon also contain omega-3 fats, a type of healthy fat that has been shown to help reduce triglyceride levels.

Studies have shown nuts, seeds, and oils that are high in linolenic acid can reduce lipid levels. Walnuts, pecans, almonds, and pistachios are high in omega-3 fats and fiber. However, keep in mind that these foods are high in calories, so you'll want to include them in moderation.

Legumes such as beans are high-protein, low-fat foods that can have a powerful impact on your lipid levels. Not only are they versatile and nutritious, but the protein they contain tends to be filling. Most legumes have a fairly neutral taste and are suitable for different dishes, including soups, salads, sides, dips, and entrées.

Dairy: Choose non-fat milk and yogurt rather whole milk. Cheese is generally high in saturated fat, but small portions of low-fat cheese such as mozzarella are healthy choices. Single-serve cheese slices or sticks work well, especially as a quick snack.

Dessert: Avoid sweets made with full-fat milk, butter, and sugar. Many packaged cakes, cookies, and snacks contain trans fats, which can raise "bad" cholesterol and lower "good" cholesterol. Instead, bake your own low-cholesterol desserts using fruit, egg whites, and oats.

Beverages: Herbal tea, especially green tea, may help lower cholesterol. Citrus juice may also have a beneficial impact on cholesterol levels. Alcoholic beverages, especially mixed drinks and cocktails, can be sources of extra calories and sugar, and increase triglycerides.

Recommended Timing

In 2019, researchers reviewed the findings from the Nutrition and Health Survey in Taiwan to see if the timing of meals had any specific impact on cholesterol levels.

The research indicated people who ate more at night may have higher LDL cholesterol levels than people who ate most of their food during the day.

When these individuals consumed what would normally be their late-day calories earlier in the day instead, they had lower cholesterol levels.

Another group of researchers looked at whether skipping meals had an effect on cholesterol levels. The research found people who skipped breakfast had higher LDL cholesterol, and people who skipped dinner had more triglycerides and a higher ratio of total and HDL cholesterol.

Cooking Tips

As you're preparing meals, you can reduce the fat content of meat by:

• Selecting lean cuts of meat with no visible fat

• Trimming remaining fat or gristle from meat and removing the skin before serving

• Grilling, broiling, or roasting meat rather than frying it with high-fat butter or oil

With fruits and vegetables, avoid adding salt, sugar, butter, or canola oil, which are high in trans fats. To avoid diminishing their nutritional power, avoid adding any sweet sauces, fat, or grease to beans and legumes.

Instead, add flavor with spices. Aside from being tasty, many popular herbs and spices have properties that can change how LDL cholesterol interacts with free radicals—particles that can make the molecules in LDL unstable, causing inflammation and further impacting your cardiovascular health. The antioxidants in some fresh herbs and spices have been shown to prevent these damaging interactions. Garlic is another healthy and versatile option for savory meals that can help lower cholesterol and triglyceride levels.

When baking, try adding ginger, allspice, and cinnamon, all of which are high in antioxidants. Instead of making baked goods using lard, butter, or oil, try using substitutes like applesauce, banana, or even avocado.

Modifications

Again, the diet recommended for you will be tailored to your condition and overall health profile. Your doctor may suggest a more strict plan for you, for example, if you have several compounding risk factors at play.

Even still, sometimes changing how you eat may not be enough to lower your cholesterol. Adding other lifestyle modifications like increasing your physical activity and losing weight may also prove insufficient.

If your levels are still high on a low cholesterol diet, your doctor may prescribe statins, medications that would be taken as you continue on with your diet for high cholesterol.

Considerations

If you're planning to make changes to your diet, it's important to consider all the different parts of your life that might be affected. Your lifestyle, responsibilities, and preferences also influence your ability to make (and stick to) the changes you make.

General Nutrition

Compared to diets that heavily restrict which foods you can eat, a diet for high cholesterol can be quite varied and balanced. Fresh produce, lean meats, and low-fat dairy are all approved on this plan and part of a healthy diet for anyone.

Many of the foods you may want to avoid or limit on a low-cholesterol diet are high in fat, sugar, and calories. Choosing not to include these foods in your diet (or having them only in moderation) can have health benefits beyond managing cholesterol, such as helping you lose weight or lower your blood pressure.

Flexibility

Though you may need to expand your typical shopping list and modify some favorite recipes, the wide range of foods that are appropriate on a diet for high cholesterol make the plan quite flexible.

Many restaurant menus highlight heart-healthy or low-fat selections, which may be appropriate. You can also ask to make simple swaps like a whole-grain wrap instead of a bun, or grilled chicken instead of fried.

Dietary Restrictions

If you're not sure how to make your dietary needs and preferences work with a low-cholesterol diet, you may want to talk with a registered dietitian or nutritionist. They can guide you through creating a lipid-lowering meal plan.

Such advice can be particularly helpful if you are also managing a gastrointestinal concern that is worsened by fiber/roughage or you need to avoid gluten (millet, teff, and quinoa are choices that are safe and packed with fiber).

Side Effects

By itself, a cholesterol-lowering diet shouldn't have any side effects. Whenever you make changes to how you eat, it's possible you will experience temporary bowel symptoms such as constipation, but these are usually temporary and get better as you adjust.

If you are starting a cholesterol-lowering drug as well, remember that any side effects you experience could also be the result of your medication. For example, muscle pain and weakness are common side effects of statins. Speak to your doctor about anything you're experiencing that is of concern.

General Health

The foods recommended to manage high cholesterol offer a myriad of other health benefits. Two in particular—helping you maintain a healthy weight and improving your energy—

can make other changes, like exercising more, easier to adopt.

This can obviously help your cholesterol-lowering efforts, but it will also help reduce your risk of issues beyond cardiovascular ones, including cancer.

5-Day Meal Plan To Lower Cholesterol

Need ideas to get started on the best food plan for lowering cholesterol?

That's what this 5-day meal plan is all about. What's more, many of the tips and recipes are so simple that even noncooks will feel, "I can do this!"

Enjoy to your heart's content.

DAY 1

Breakfast

• Oatmeal with Fresh Berries and Nonfat Milk or Soymilk

Oats are high in cholesterol-lowering soluble fiber. So are berries, all berries – blackberries, raspberries, strawberries, blueberries. How tasty!

• Tea or Coffee, If Desired

If you'd like, add a little nonfat milk or soymilk and/or a packet of sugar substitute. Good, proven-to-be-safe choices are sucralose (Splenda) and stevia (many brands are available, such as Truvia and SweetLeaf)

Mid-Morning Snack (If you're hungry)

- Baby Carrots and Broccoli with Greek Yogurt Dip

To make this dip, combine in a small mixing bowl ¾ cup plain nonfat Greek yogurt, 1 minced garlic clove, 2 tablespoons chives, 1 tablespoon lemon juice, and a few grinds of black pepper. Use leftovers as a creamy, tangy, totally healthy topping for your baked potato on Day 2.

Lunch

- Sweet Potato with a Dollop of Dijon Mustard (Low-Sodium)

No time to bake a sweet potato? No worries! Microwave it. Simply pierce the skin 5 or 6 times. Then nuke for about 6 minutes, depending on the size of your sweet potato, rotating halfway through. It's done when the skin puffs to a crisp finish and is soft to the touch. The flesh should be sweet and pillowy.

• Big Salad of Romaine Lettuce, Red Onions, and Cherry Tomatoes Tossed with Aged Balsamic Vinegar and Grilled Tofu Cubes

Mid-Afternoon Snack (If you're hungry)

• A Big, Crisp Apple

Dinner

• Big Salad of Baby Greens Tossed with Pritikin's Tuscan Sunshine Italian Dressing

Unlike many other salad dressings, Pritikin's dressings are genuinely low in added sodium, sugars, and fats, and bursting with flavor from savory ingredients like ginger, herbs, and mustards. They're developed by Pritikin's chefs right in the kitchen at the Pritikin Longevity Center.

• Salmon with Sweet Chili Sauce

• Garlic-Roasted Brussels Sprouts

Vegetables are great sources of soluble fiber, with Brussels sprouts topping the list. Use the leftovers as a wonderfully "meaty" addition to tomorrow afternoon's green salad.

Dessert (If you're hungry)

• Vanilla Yogurt (Nonfat, No-Sugar-Added, 1 Cup) with Fresh Raspberries

DAY 2

Breakfast

• Egg-White Omelet with Fresh Salsa and Chopped Green Onions

Even simpler than making an omelet: Cook your eggs in the microwave. Lightly spray the inside of a microwaveable bowl with oil spray like Pam. Scramble your egg whites in the bowl. Add veggies, black pepper, or no-salt-added seasoning like Pritikin All-Purpose Seasoning. Nuke, covered, for about 1 to 2 minutes, depending on the heat of your microwave.

• Half of Cantaloupe Filled with Cottage Cheese (Fat-Free, Low-Sodium)

A good brand choice for fat-free, low-sodium cottage cheese is Friendship. There are also store brands.

• Coffee or Tea, If Desired

If you'd like, add a little nonfat milk or soymilk and/or a packet of Splenda or stevia.

Mid-Morning Snack (If you're hungry)

- Pear

Keep a big bowl full of fresh fruit – apples, bananas, pears, grapefruits, tangerines, grapes, and more – on your kitchen counter. Recent research10 found that people who have bowls of fruit on their kitchen counters weigh significantly less than people who do not.

Lunch

- Big Salad of Baby Spinach and Roasted Brussels Sprouts (saved from last night's dinner)

- "Homemade" Barley Soup for the NonCook

Yes, you can do this! In the freezer section of the grocery store, pick up a box of Tabatchnick Barley and Mushroom Soup – Low Sodium. While it's heating up on the stove, toss in ½ to 1 cup of sliced fresh mushrooms and ½ cup chopped celery. Ladle your soup into a bowl and top with freshly diced green onions, if desired. So gourmet! So easy!

Mid-Afternoon Snack (If you're hungry)

• Big Handful of Grapes

Fresh fruit every day helps your heart, a large, 500,000-person study11 recently found. Those who ate fresh fruit every day had about one-third reduced risk of dying from a heart attack compared to those who rarely or never ate fruit.

Dinner

• Meatless Burger Topped with Slices of Roasted Red Pepper

Veggie patties have only about half the calories of red meat patties, and 0 artery-clogging saturated fat. Good low-sodium, high-soluble-fiber choices are Engine 2 Pinto Habanero and Tuscan Kale White Bean, available at Whole Foods Markets.

Top your burger with slices of roasted red bell pepper. So smoky and savory! Roast 5 or 6 peppers at a time so that you can use them throughout the week on salads, in soups, or as a side dish.

Here's how: Preheat your broiler to high and roast your whole peppers under the broiler on an aluminum-wrapped tray for 15 to 20 minutes, turning every 5 minutes as their skins darken to black. Remove. Cool. Then remove skins, stems, and seeds, and slice. Refrigerate leftovers.

• Baked Potato with the Greek Yogurt Dip Saved from Yesterday's Mid-Morning Snack

Or top your baked potato with nonfat sour cream and chives.

Dessert (If you're hungry)

• Passion Fruit

DAY 3

Breakfast

• Homemade Muesli

Grate 1 apple or pear. Mix with ¼ cup of dry rolled oats and ½ cup of nonfat, plain Greek yogurt. Allow to stand for 15 minutes or refrigerate overnight. Stir in a packet of Splenda or stevia, and top with a tablespoon of flaxseeds.

• Coffee or Tea, If Desired

If you'd like, add a little nonfat milk or soymilk and/or a packet of Splenda or stevia.

Mid-Morning Snack (If you're hungry)

• Navel Orange or 2 to 3 Tangerines

Lunch

• Asian Edamame Salad

This salad is "heavy" enough to serve as a one-dish meal. It also packs some nice tang, nuttiness, and crunch. You can often find edamame (soybeans) in both the refrigerated and frozen sections of supermarkets.

For the dressing, whisk together a tablespoon of rice vinegar, a pinch of wasabi, and a teaspoon of freshly grated ginger. Toss with ¾ cup edamame, ¼ chopped cucumber, ¼ cup chopped celery, and a handful of sliced radishes.

• Steamed Asparagus

Mid-Afternoon Snack (If you're hungry)

• Corn on the Cob

Microwave, husk and all, for 3 to 5 minutes. Alternatively, microwave a husked ear of corn by wetting a paper towel and wringing it out. Wrap the ear in the moist towel and cook for 3 to 5 minutes.

Dinner

• Trout Fillets with Mango Salsa

Serves 2.

Season two 4-ounce trout fillets with Pritikin Fish Seasoning or other salt-free seasonings, such as lemon pepper. Place in a 350-degree oven and bake till meat is opaque and flakes easily with a fork, about 20 minutes.

Top with Mango Salsa. What flavor! To make it, combine 2 cups chopped mango, 1 cup chopped cucumber, 1 cup halved cherry tomatoes, ¼ cup finely chopped cilantro leaves, 2 tablespoons of lime juice, and half of a very finely diced jalapeno, seeds removed. Leftovers make superb toppings for veggie burgers or other fish, such as salmon and tilapia.

- Big Salad with Kale and Sliced Apple
- Super-Simple White Bean Soup

Lightly mist a heavy nonstick pot with oil spray. Over high heat, sauté a half-pound of diced carrots till they start to brown, stirring constantly. Add 4 cloves of minced garlic, a teaspoon of salt-free Italian seasoning, and a pinch of red pepper flakes (more if you like it hotter). Stir for another minute. Add a 15-ounce can of no-salt-added diced tomatoes and 1-1/2 cups of water. Simmer till carrots are tender, about 10 minutes. Stir in a 15-ounce can of white beans (no salt added) and heat through. Finish with black pepper. Refrigerate or freeze leftovers.

Dessert (If you're hungry)

• Chocolate Nonfat Frozen Yogurt (1/2 cup)

A good brand choice is Stonyfield Nonfat After Dark Chocolate. Do keep your serving to a half cup. Any more and you're swallowing a lot of added sugar.

DAY 4

Breakfast

• Tofu Scramble

The night before, press 4 to 6 ounces of extra-firm tofu to drain water. In a small bowl, combine a little balsamic vinegar, dry oregano, and minced garlic. Pour over tofu. Marinate overnight. Come morning, sauté sliced onions and green bell pepper in a nonstick skillet until softened. Add tofu, crumbling it into bite-sized pieces. Cook till slightly browned, about 5 minutes.

- 1/2 Whole-Grain Bagel, Toasted

Top with nonfat ricotta cheese and sliced strawberries

- Coffee or Tea, If Desired

If you'd like, add a little nonfat milk or soymilk and/or a packet of Splenda or stevia.

Mid-Morning Snack (If you're hungry)

- Banana

Lunch

- Toasted Barley Salad with Mixed Veggies

Dry-toasting barley adds a nutty taste and helps the barley retain its chewy texture.

Place ½ cup of pearl barley in a heavy, large saucepan. Cook over medium heat until pale golden, shaking pan occasionally, about 10 minutes. Add 1-1/2 cups of low-sodium vegetable broth to pan. Bring to boil. Reduce heat to medium-low. Cover and simmer till barley is tender and broth is absorbed, about 35 minutes. Uncover. Let barley cool.

Toss cooked barley with romaine lettuce, sweet onions, fresh mushrooms, and red bell pepper, all chopped. Mix in a zesty dressing that's low in fat, sugar, and sodium

• Vanilla Yogurt (Nonfat, No-Sugar-Added, 1 Cup) with Fresh Blueberries

Mid-Afternoon Snack (If you're hungry)

• Celery Sticks with Pineapple Hummus Dip

Dinner

• Black Bean Soft Tacos

Light mist with oil spray a small, nonstick pan. Saute 1 diced onion until soft, about 3 minutes. Stir in a teaspoon of minced garlic and a teaspoon of chili powder. Add one 15-ounce can of no-salt-added black beans, including liquid. Simmer for 5 minutes. Spoon about a third of your beans into 2 warm corn tortillas. Top with shredded cabbage and fresh lime juice. Save remaining beans as a delish addition to your next green salad.

• Roasted Red Peppers and Browned Onions

Use the extra peppers you roasted on Day 2 and combine with a big, sliced onion that you've sautéed on the stove. Season with black pepper and garlic powder.

Dessert (If you're hungry)

• Watermelon Cooler

Combine 2 cups of chopped watermelon, 1 cup of crushed ice, ½ cup of chopped cucumber, a few fresh mint leaves, and 1 tablespoon of fresh lime juice in a blender. Blend till smooth.

DAY 5

Breakfast

• Oatmeal with Fresh Berries and Nonfat Milk or Soymilk

Whatever type of oatmeal you buy, always read the Ingredient List to make sure there is no added sugar or sodium. Instant oatmeal (especially single-serving packets) are often high in added sugars and sodium.

• Coffee or Tea, If Desired

If you'd like, add a little nonfat milk or soymilk and/or a packet of Splenda or stevia.

Mid-Morning Snack (If you're hungry)

• Salad in a Second

At the market, pick up bags of pre-washed, pre-cut salad greens and veggies. When hunger hits, just pour the whole bag into a big bowl and toss with really good aged balsamic vinegar or a savory dressing low in fat, sugar, and salt

Lunch

• So-Easy Veggie and Red Bean Soup

At the market, buy a bag of Mann's Power Blend Veggies. It's 10 ounces of shredded, ready-to-use veggies full of cholesterol-reducing soluble fiber, such as Brussels sprouts, Napa cabbage, broccoli, carrots, and kale. Pour the whole bag into a stockpot along with a can of red beans (no salt added), 1 to 1.5 quarts of low-sodium vegetable broth, minced garlic, and 2 teaspoons of salt-free seasoning like Pritikin's All-Purpose Seasoning. Bring to a boil, then simmer for about 20 minutes. That's it! Delicious homemade soup.

Can't find Mann's? Your supermarket may carry its own brand of assorted, shredded veggies. One good choice is Trader Joe's Cruciferous Crunch (Brussels sprouts, kale, broccoli, and cabbage varieties).

Brown Rice

Don't want to spend 40 minutes cooking brown rice? You don't have to anymore. Many stores carry freshly cooked brown rice (usually in the deli section) or single-serving bowls in the rice/pasta section that need just 60 to 90 minutes in a microwave. Just make sure you're getting pure rice (no sodium or other ingredients in the Ingredient List).

Mid-Afternoon Snack (If you're hungry)

• Baked Sweet Potato with Nonfat, Plain Greek Yogurt Swirled In

Dinner

• Pritikin Caesar Salad

• Vegetarian Chili

Dessert (If you're hungry)

• Cup of Fresh Pineapple with 2 Tablespoons Thinly Sliced Fresh Basil

LOW CHOLESTEROL DIET RECIPES

Trying a low cholesterol-friendly recipes is a great way to explore new flavors and find new favorite dishes while looking after your health. In this part are nourishing low cholesterol diet recipes for healthy living.

Parmesan Potato Pancakes

Preparation time

22 minutes

Ingredients

- 2 cups leftover mashed potatoes

- 2 tablespoons chopped fresh chives or green onions

- 1 large egg white

- 1/4 cup seasoned breadcrumbs, divided

- 2 tablespoons grated fresh Parmesan cheese

- 2 teaspoons olive oil, divided

Instructions

1. Combine potatoes, chives, egg white, and 2 tablespoons breadcrumbs in a large bowl.

2. Combine 2 tablespoons breadcrumbs and cheese on a small plate.

3. Divide the potato mixture into 8 equal (1/4-cup) portions; dredge in breadcrumb mixture, shaping each portion into a 1/4-inch-thick patty.

4. Heat 1 teaspoon oil in large nonstick skillet.

5. Add 4 patties; cook 3-4 minutes on each side or until golden.

6. Repeat with 1 teaspoon oil and remaining 4 patties.

7. Serve pancakes hot with applesauce and low-fat sour cream.

Penne with eggplant caponata

Preparation time

30 minutes

INGREDIENTS

- 2 tablespoons olive oil

- 1 onion, chopped

- 2 garlic cloves, finely chopped

- 1 large eggplant (about 500g), cut into 2cm cubes

- 2 x 400g cans chopped tomatoes

- 2 teaspoons caster sugar

- 1/2 cup (60g) pitted green olives

- 1/3 cup (65g) drained capers

- 2 tablespoons chopped fl at-leaf parsley

- 400g penne rigate

* 2 tablespoons freshly grated parmesan (or vegetarian hard cheese)

Instructions

1. Heat oil in a pan over medium heat.

2. Add the onion and garlic and gently cook, stirring, for 5 minutes or until light golden. Increase heat to high, add eggplant and cook, stirring, for 2-3 minutes until golden, then add tomatoes, sugar and a little salt and pepper.

3. Bring to the boil, then simmer over low heat for 15 minutes or until the eggplant is cooked and sauce thickens.

4. Stir in the olives, capers and parsley.

5. Meanwhile, cook the pasta according to packet instructions.

6. Drain well, then toss with sauce and serve with parmesan.

Chicken with cannellini bean and tomato sauce

Preparation time

30 minutes

INGREDIENTS

- Olive oil spray

- 1 small red onion, finely chopped

- 2 garlic cloves, crushed

- 1 teaspoon crushed red chilli

- 1 x 400g can no-added-salt chopped tomatoes

- 1 x 400g can no-added-salt cannellini beans, rinsed, drained

- 2 teaspoons salted baby capers, rinsed, drained, coarsely chopped

- 2 tablespoons chopped fresh continental parsley

- 2 (about 250g each) Lilydale Free Range Chicken Breasts, halved horizontally

- Steamed green round beans, to serve

Instructions

1. Heat a saucepan over medium-low heat.

2. Spray with olive oil spray to grease.

3. Add the onion and cook, stirring occasionally, for 5 minutes or until soft.

4. Add the garlic and chilli, and cook, stirring, for 1 minute or until aromatic.

5. Add the tomato. Increase heat to high and bring to the boil.

6. Reduce heat to low and simmer for 5 minutes.

7. Add the cannellini beans and capers, and simmer for 5 minutes or until the mixture thickens slightly.

8. Season with pepper.

9. Stir in half the parsley.

10. Meanwhile, heat a large non-stick frying pan over high heat.

11. Spray with olive oil spray.

12. Add the chicken and cook for 2-3 minutes each side or until golden and cooked through.

13. Divide the chicken among serving plates.

14. Top with the cannellini bean mixture and remaining parsley.

15. Serve with steamed green beans.

Chilled Avocado Soup

Preparation time

2 hours 25 minutes

Ingredients

- 4 ripe avocados, pitted and peeled

- 6 tbsp fresh lemon juice

- 3 cups low-fat plain yogurt

- 3 cups chicken broth

- 4 large fresh basil leaves, slivered

- ¼ tsp black pepper, freshly ground

- pinch of salt

- 4 large fresh basil leaves, for garnish

- 4 radishes, finely chopped, for garnish

Instructions

1. Set aside half of one to the avocados and place it in a small bowl.

2. Sprinkle it with 1 tablespoon of the lemon juice, cover loosely, and refrigerate.

3. Coarsely chop the remaining 3 ½ avocados, and place them in a large bowl.

4. Add the remaining 5 tablespoon lemon juice, and toss.

5. Add the yogurt, stock, slivered basil, pepper, and salt to the chopped avocados, and stir well.

6. Transfer the mixture to a food processor and process until fairly smooth, scraping down the sides of the bowl if necessary.

7. Do not puree entirely.

8. A bit of texture should remain.

9. Remove the mixture to another bowl, cover, and chill for 2 hours.

10. Sliver the basil for the garnish right before serving.

11. Dice the remaining avocado half.

12. Divide the soup among individual soup bowls.

13. Sprinkle the portions evenly with the diced avocado, and top with the radishes and slivered basil, if desired.

Sugar-Free Apple Pie

Preparation time

1 hour 38 minutes

Ingredients

- 2 tsp tapioca or cornstarch flour

- 1 tsp cinnamon or nutmeg, ground

- ½ cup apple juice cider

- 4 cup green apples, sliced

- 20 oz pie crust dough, prepared

- 1 egg yolk

- 1 tbsp milk

- all-purpose flour, for dusting

Instructions

1. Preheat your oven to 325F and grease a 9-inch pie tin.

2. Assemble the filling by combining the tapioca or cornstarch flour, cinnamon or nutmeg, apple juice cider, and green apples together.

3. Mix until evenly incorporated and then set aside.

4. Dust both your rolling pin and working area with flour, and roll out 1 disc of dough until you achieve roughly ½-inch thickness.

5. Transfer the dough onto your pie tin and ensure to leave excess dough hanging on the sides of the pie tin.

6. Pour your filling onto your pie tin. Set aside.

7. Repeat steps 3 with your remaining disc of dough, but this time to cover the pie.

8. Seal edges and make a few slits in top.

9. Prepare your egg wash. Beat together egg yolk & milk.

10. Brush this around & on top of your pie.

11. Transfer to the oven and bake for roughly 40 minutes.

12. Then, increase your oven temperature to 400F.

13. Broil the crush until golden, roughly around 10 minutes

14. Once baked, transfer the pie onto cooling racks & allow to cool completely

15. Portion accordingly & serve

Starbucks Oatmeal With Fresh Blueberries

Preparation time

15 minutes

Ingredients

- 1 ⅓ cup water

- ¼ tsp cinnamon

- 2 tsp mild honey

- ⅔ cup oatmeal

- ⅓ cup fresh blueberries

- ½ tsp orange zest, grated

- ½ cup almond milk

Instructions

1. Boil water in a medium-size saucepan, then stir in the salt, cinnamon, honey and oatmeal.

2. Reduce the heat to simmering and cook uncovered for five minutes.

3. Stir in the orange zest and milk, then simmer for five more minutes or until the oatmeal is thick and creamy.

4. Cover the oatmeal and let cool for five minutes, then serve topped with fresh blueberries.

Zingy salmon & brown rice salad

Preparation time

40 minutes

Ingredients

- 200g brown basmati rice

- 200g frozen soya beans , defrosted

- 2 salmon fillets

- 1 cucumber , diced

- small bunch spring onions , sliced

- small bunch coriander , roughly chopped

- zest and juice 1 lime

- 1 red chilli , diced, deseeded if you like

- 4 tsp light soy sauce

Instructions

1. Cook the rice following pack instructions and 3 mins before it's done, add the soya beans.

2. Drain and cool under cold running water.

3. Meanwhile, put the salmon on a plate, then microwave on High for 3 mins or until cooked through.

4. Allow to cool slightly, remove the skin with a fork, then flake.

5. Gently fold the cucumber, spring onions, coriander and salmon into the rice and beans.

6. In a separate bowl, mix the lime zest and juice, chilli and soy, then pour over the rice before serving.

Vegetable tagine with chickpeas & raisins

Preparation time

10 minutes

Ingredients

- 2 tbsp olive oil

- 2 onions , chopped

- ½ tsp each ground cinnamon , coriander and cumin

- 2 large courgettes , cut into chunks

- 2 chopped tomatoes

- 400g can chickpea , rinsed and drained

- 4 tbsp raisin

- 425ml vegetable stock

- 300g frozen pea

- chopped coriander , to serve

Instructions

1. Heat the oil in a pan, then fry the onions for 5 mins until soft.

2. Stir in the spices.

3. Add the courgettes, tomatoes, chickpeas, raisins and stock, then bring to the boil.

4. Cover and simmer for 10 mins.

5. Stir in the peas and cook for 5 mins more. Sprinkle with coriander, to serve.

Savoy cabbage with almonds

Preparation time

25 minutes

Ingredients

- 1 Savoy cabbage , finely sliced

- 25g butter

- 1 tbsp olive oil

- 1 garlic clove , sliced

- 1 rosemary sprig, leaves finely chopped

- 100g blanched almond

Instructions

1. Steam or microwave the cabbage until just cooked.

2. Melt the butter with the oil in a large frying pan or wok, then add the garlic, rosemary and almonds.

3. Cook, stirring the almonds for about 2 mins or until they start to brown.

4. Tip onto a plate.

5. Add the cabbage to the pan, stir in the leftover buttery juices, then return the almond mixture to the pan.

6. Season well and tip into a serving dish.

Noodles with turkey, green beans & hoisin

Preparation time

25 minutes

Ingredients

- 100g ramen noodles

- 100g green beans , halved

- 3 tbsp hoisin sauce

- juice 1 lime

- 1 tbsp chilli sauce

- 1 tbsp vegetable oil

- 250g turkey mince

- 2 garlic cloves , chopped

- 6 spring onions , sliced diagonally

Instructions

1. Boil the noodles following pack instructions, adding the green beans for the final 2 mins.

2. Drain and set aside.

3. In a small bowl, mix together the hoisin, lime juice and chilli sauce.

4. In a wok or frying pan, heat the oil, then fry the mince until nicely browned.

5. Add the garlic and fry for 1 min more.

6. Stir in the hoisin mixture and cook for a few mins more until sticky.

7. Finally, stir in the noodles, beans and half the spring onions to heat through.

8. Scatter over the remaining spring onions to serve.

Trout en papillote

Preparation time

30 minutes

Ingredients

- 2 large carrots , cut into batons

- 3 celery sticks, cut into batons

- 1 tbsp olive oil

- ½ tsp sugar

- 6 tbsp white wine vinegar

- 4 x 175g trout fillets

- basil leaves

- juice 1 lemon

Instructions

1. Heat oven to 190C/fan 170C/gas 5.

2. Put the carrots and celery in a pan with the oil, sugar, wine, salt and pepper.

3. Bring to the boil, tightly cover, then cook for 10 mins until the vegetables are tender. Cool.

4. Cut four large sheets of baking parchment, about 35cm square.

5. Divide the vegetables between them and top each with a trout fillet.

6. Scatter a few basil leaves and a little lemon juice over each, then season the fish with a little salt and pepper.

7. Fold the paper in half and double fold all round to seal in the fish, a bit like a pasty.

8. Put the parcels on two baking sheets and bake for 15-20 mins (depending on the thickness of the fish).

9. Serve in their paper with some steamed new potatoes.

Salmon & spinach with tartare cream

Preparation time

15 minutes

Ingredients

- 1 tsp sunflower or vegetable oil

- 2 skinless salmon fillets

- 250g bag spinach

- 2 tbsp reduced-fat crème fraîche

- juice ½ lemon

- 1 tsp caper, drained

- 2 tbsp flat-leaf parsley, chopped

• lemon wedges, to serve

Instructions

1. Heat the oil in a pan, season the salmon on both sides, then fry for 4 mins each side until golden and the flesh flakes easily.

2. Leave to rest on a plate while you cook the spinach.

3. Tip the leaves into the hot pan, season well, then cover and leave to wilt for 1 min, stirring once or twice.

4. Spoon the spinach onto plates, then top with the salmon.

5. Gently heat the crème fraîche in the pan with a squeeze of the lemon juice, the capers and parsley, then season to taste.

6. Be careful not to let it boil.

7. Spoon the sauce over the fish, then serve with lemon wedges.

Indian Winter Soup

Preparation time

45 minutes

Ingredients

- 100g pearl barley

- 2 tbsp vegetable oil

- ½ tsp brown mustard seeds

- 1 tsp cumin seeds

- 2 green chillies, deseeded and finely chopped

- 1 bay leaf

- 2 cloves

- 1 small cinnamon stick

- ½ tsp ground turmeric

- 1 large onion, chopped

- 2 garlic cloves, finely chopped

- 1 parsnip, cut into chunks

- 200g butternut squash, cut into chunks

- 200g sweet potato, cut into chunks

- 1 tsp paprika

- 1 tsp ground coriander

- 225g red lentils

- 2 tomatoes, chopped

- small bunch coriander, chopped

- 1 tsp grated ginger

- 1 tsp lemon juice

Instructions

1. Rinse the pearl barley and cook following pack instructions.

2. When it is tender, drain and set aside.

3. Meanwhile, heat the oil in a deep, heavy-bottomed pan.

4. Fry the mustard seeds, cumin seeds, chillies, bay leaf, cloves, cinnamon and turmeric until fragrant and the seeds start to crackle.

5. Tip in the onion and garlic, then cook for 5-8 mins until soft. Stir in the parsnip, butternut and sweet potato and mix thoroughly, making sure the vegetables are fully coated with the oil and spices.

6. Sprinkle in the paprika, ground coriander and seasoning, and stir again.

7. Add the lentils, pearl barley, tomatoes and 1.7 litres water.

8. Bring to the boil then turn down and simmer until the vegetables are tender.

9. When the lentils are almost cooked, stir in the chopped coriander, ginger and lemon juice.

The ultimate makeover: Fish pie

Preparation time

1 hour 20 minutes

Ingredients

- 500ml semi-skimmed milk

- 3 tbsp cornflour

- 100g cooked prawns in their shells

- several thyme sprigs, preferably lemon thyme

- 2 bay leaves

- 1 garlic clove , thinly sliced

- 750g new potatoes , such as Charlotte (no need to peel)

- 1 medium leek , thinly sliced (175g prepared weight)

- 400g skinned haddock fillet

- 350g skinned salmon fillet

- 175g skinned smoked haddock fillet

- 125g tub low-fat soft cheese with garlic & herbs

- 2 tbsp finely chopped parsley

- 2 tbsp olive oil

- 2 tbsp snipped chives

Instructions

1. Mix 3 tbsp of the milk into the cornflour and set aside.

2. Pour the rest of the milk into a saucepan.

3.   Shell the prawns, reserve the meat, then drop the shells and heads (wash them first if necessary) into the milk along with the thyme sprigs, bay leaves, garlic and a grind of pepper.

4.   Bring to a boil, then remove from the heat and leave to infuse for 20 mins.

5. Meanwhile, put the potatoes into a large pan of water, bring to the boil and simmer for 20 mins until tender.

6. Drain.

7. Steam the sliced leek for 3 mins, then remove from the heat and set aside.

8. Strain the infused milk through a sieve into a large shallow sauté pan.

9. Lay all the fish fillets (not the prawns) in the milk.

10. Bring to a boil, then lower the heat and simmer gently for 3 mins.

11. Remove from the heat and leave, covered, for 5 mins.

12. Use a slotted spoon to transfer all the fish to a dish and leave to cool slightly.

13. Heat oven to 200C/180C fan/gas 6.

14. Stir the slackened cornflour, then stir it into the hot milk in the sauté pan.

15. Return the pan to the heat and stir until thickened.

16. Briefly stir in the soft cheese, remove from the heat, then add the parsley and season with black pepper.

17. Stir in any liquid that has drained from the fish.

18. Break the fish into big pieces as you lay them in a 2-litre ovenproof dish so that the different varieties are evenly distributed.

19. Scatter over the prawns and leek, then season with pepper.

20. Pour the sauce over and give a few gentle stirs to evenly distribute the sauce and combine everything without breaking up the fish.

21. Using a large fork, crush the potatoes by breaking them up (not mashing them) into chunky pieces.

22. Mix in the oil, chives and a grind of black pepper.

23. Spoon the potato crush over the fish.

24. Sit the dish on a baking sheet and bake for 25-30 mins, or until the sauce is bubbling and the potatoes golden.

25. Alternatively, make the dish completely, refrigerate it for several hrs or overnight, then bake at the same temperature as above for 45 mins.

Seeded Oatcakes

Preparation time

30 minutes

Ingredients

- 50g butter

- 100g medium oatmeal

- 100g plain flour , plus extra for dusting

- 1 tsp bicarbonate of soda

- 2 tsp poppy seed

- 2 tbsp sesame seed

Instructions

1. Heat oven to 200C/180C fan/gas 6. Melt the butter in a small pan, then allow to cool slightly.

2. Tip all the dry ingredients into a bowl, with ½ tsp salt, then pour in the butter.

3. Add 5-6 tbsp boiling water and combine to make a firm dough.

4. Turn out the dough onto a lightly floured surface, then roll out until about 0.5cm thick.

5. Cut into small squares, then bake for 12-15 mins until golden.

6. Leave to cool for a few mins, then transfer to a wire rack and cool completely.

Devilled tofu kebabs

Preparation time

35 minutes

Ingredients

- 8 shallots or button onions

- 8 small new potatoes

- 2 tbsp tomato purée

- 2 tbsp light soy sauce

- 1 tbsp sunflower oil

- 1 tbsp clear honey

- 1 tbsp wholegrain mustard

- 300g firm smoked tofu , cubed

- 1 courgette , peeled and sliced

- 1 red pepper , deseeded and diced

Instructions

1. Put the shallots or button onions in a bowl, cover with boiling water and set aside for 5 mins.

2. Cook the potatoes in a pan of boiling water for 7 mins until tender.

3. Drain and pat dry.

4. Put tomato purée, soy sauce, oil, honey, mustard and seasoning in a bowl, then mix well.

5. Toss the tofu in the marinade. Set aside for at least 10 mins.

6. Heat the grill.

7. Drain and peel shallots or onions, then cook in boiling water for 3 mins.

8. Drain well.

9. Thread the tofu, shallots, potatoes, courgette and pepper on to 8 x 20cm skewers.

10. Grill for 10 mins, turning frequently and brushing with remaining marinade before serving.

Edamame & chilli dip with crudités

Preparation time

15 minutes

Ingredients

- 300g frozen soya bean

- 150g low-fat natural yogurt

- 1 red chilli , chopped

- juice 1 lime

- 1 garlic clove , crushed

- 1 red onion , finely chopped

- handful coriander , chopped

- halved radishes , sticks of carrots, celery and peppers, to serve

Instructions

1. Cook the soya beans in boiling salted water for 4 mins.

2. Drain and cool under cold running water.

3. Blitz with the yogurt, chopped red chilli, lime juice and crushed garlic clove until smooth.

4. Fold in the finely chopped red onion and a handful chopped coriander.

5. Serve with halved radishes and sticks of carrots, celery and peppers.

6. The dip will keep covered in the fridge for up to 3 days.

Spiced quinoa with almonds & feta

Preparation time

25 minutes

Ingredients

- 1 tbsp olive oil

- 1 tsp ground coriander

- ½ tsp turmeric

- 300g quinoa , rinsed

- 50g toasted flaked almonds

- 100g feta cheese , crumbled

- handful parsley , roughly chopped

- juice ½ lemon

Instructions

1. Heat the oil in a large pan. Add the spices, then fry for a min or so until fragrant.

2. Add the quinoa, then fry for a further min until you can hear gentle popping sounds.

3. Stir in 600ml boiling water, then gently simmer for 10-15 mins until the water has evaporated and the quinoa grains have a white 'halo' around them.

4. Allow to cool slightly, then stir through the other ingredients.

5. Serve warm or cold.

Summer vegetable curry

Preparation time

45 minutes

Ingredients

- 1-2 tbsp red Thai curry paste (depending on taste)

- 500ml low-sodium vegetable stock

- 2 onions , chopped

- 1 aubergine , diced

- 75g red lentil

- 200ml can reduced-fat coconut milk

- 2 red or yellow peppers , deseeded and cut into wedges

- 140g frozen pea

- 100g bag baby spinach , roughly chopped

- brown basmati rice and mango chutney, to serve

Instructions

1. Heat the curry paste in a large non-stick saucepan with a splash of the stock.

2. Add the onions and fry for 5 mins until starting to soften.

3. Stir in the aubergine and cook for a further 5 mins – add a little more stock if starting to stick.

4. Add the lentils, coconut milk and the rest of the stock, and simmer for 15 mins or until the lentils are tender.

5. Add the peppers and cook for 5-10 mins more.

6. Stir through the peas and spinach and cook until spinach has just wilted.

7. Serve the curry with rice and mango chutney.

Tomato, sardine & rocket

Preparation time

10 minutes

Ingredients

- a thick slice baguette

- 1 garlic clove

- 1 ripe tomato

- good-quality sardines , from a can

- rocket

Instructions

1. Toast a thick slice of baguette.

2. Cut the garlic clove in half and rub the cut side over the surface.

3. Halve the tomato and squeeze and rub the flesh over the bread.

4. Top with the sardines and rocket.

Low-fat moussaka

Preparation time

45 minutes

Ingredients

- 200g frozen sliced peppers

- 3 garlic cloves , crushed

- 200g extra-lean minced beef

- 100g red lentils

- 2 tsp dried oregano , plus extra for sprinkling

- 500ml carton passata

* 1 aubergine , sliced into 1.5cm rounds

* 4 tomatoes , sliced into 1cm rounds

* 2 tsp olive oil

* 25g parmesan , finely grated

* 170g pot 0% fat Greek yogurt

* freshly grated nutmeg

Instructions

1. Cook the peppers gently in a large non-stick pan for about 5 mins – the water from them should stop them sticking.

2. Add the garlic and cook for 1 min more, then add the beef, breaking up with a fork, and cook until brown.

3. Tip in the lentils, half the oregano, the passata and a splash of water.

4. Simmer for 15-20 mins until the lentils are tender, adding more water if you need to.

5. Meanwhile, heat the grill to Medium.

6. Arrange the aubergine and tomato slices on a non-stick baking tray and brush with the oil.

7. Sprinkle with the remaining oregano and some seasoning, then grill for 1-2 mins each side until lightly charred – you may need to do this in batches.

8. Mix half the Parmesan with the yogurt and some seasoning.

9. Divide the beef mixture between 4 small ovenproof dishes and top with the sliced aubergine and tomato.

10. Spoon over the yogurt topping and sprinkle with the extra oregano, Parmesan and nutmeg.

11. Grill for 3-4 mins until bubbling.

12. Serve with a salad, if you like.

Spiced chicken with rice & crisp red onions

Preparation time

35 minutes

Ingredients

- 2 boneless skinless chicken breasts, about 140g/5oz each

- 1 tbsp sunflower oil

- 2 tsp curry powder

- 1 large red onion , thinly sliced

- 100g basmati rice

- 1 cinnamon stick

- pinch saffron

- 1 tbsp raisins

- 85g frozen pea

- 1 tbsp chopped mint and coriander

- 4 rounded tbsp low-fat natural yogurt

Instructions

1. Heat oven to 190C/fan 170C/gas 5.

2. Brush the chicken with 1 tsp oil, then sprinkle with curry powder.

3. Toss the onion in the remaining oil.

4. Put the chicken and onions in one layer in a roasting tin.

5. Bake for 25 mins until the meat is cooked and the onions are crisp, stirring the onions halfway through the cooking time.

6. Rinse the rice, then put in a pan with the cinnamon, saffron, salt to taste and 300ml water.

7. Bring to the boil, stir once, add the raisins, cover.

8. Gently cook for 10-12 mins until the rice is tender, adding the peas halfway through.

9. Spoon the rice onto two plates, top with the chicken and scatter over the onions.

10. Stir the herbs into the yogurt and season, if you like, before serving on the side.

Crush bean, Artichoke and Red Onion

Preparation time

10 minutes

Ingredients

- 1 slice granary bread

- 1 small can haricot bean

- basil oil

- artichoke heart , from a jar

- sundried tomatoes , from a jar

- few slices red onion

Instructions

1. Toasta a slice of bread.

2. Drain the haricot beans and mash in a bowl with a little oil.

3. Season if you like.

4. Spoon over the toast and top with artichoke hearts and sundried tomatoes, a few slices red onion and a little more oil, if you like.

Crab Linguine with Chili and Parsley

Preparation time

30 minutes

Ingredients

* 400g linguine

* 4 tbsp extra-virgin olive oil

* 1 red chilli, deseeded and chopped

* 2 garlic cloves, finely chopped

* 1 whole cooked crab, picked, or about 100g/4oz brown crabmeat and 200g/7oz fresh white crabmeat

- small splash, about 5 tbsp, white wine

- small squeeze of lemon (optional)

- large handful flat-leaf parsley leaves, very finely chopped

Instructions

1. Bring a large pan of salted water to the boil and add the linguine.

2. Give it a good stir and boil for 1 min less than the pack says.

3. Stir well occasionally so it doesn't stick.

4. While the pasta cooks, gently heat 3 tbsp of olive oil with the chilli and garlic in a pan large enough to hold all the pasta comfortably.

5. Cook the chilli and garlic very gently until they start to sizzle, then turn up the heat and add the white wine.

6. Simmer everything until the wine and olive oil come together.

7. Then take off the heat and add the brown crabmeat, using a wooden spatula or spoon to mash it into the olive oil to make a thick sauce.

8. When the pasta has had its cooking time, taste a strand – it should have a very slight bite.

9. When it's ready, turn off the heat.

10. Place the sauce on a very low heat and use a pair of kitchen tongs to lift the pasta from the water into the sauce.

11. Off the heat, add the white crabmeat and parsley to the pasta with a sprinkling of sea salt.

12. Stir everything together really well, adding a drop of pasta water if it's starting to get claggy.

13. Taste for seasoning and, if it needs a slight lift, add a small squeeze of lemon.

14. Serve immediately twirled into pasta bowls and drizzled with the remaining oil.

Spaghetti with Sadine

Preparation time

20 minutes

Ingredients

- 400g spaghetti

- 1 tbsp olive oil

- 2 garlic cloves , crushed

- pinch chilli flakes

- 227g can chopped tomato

- x cans skinless and boneless sardines in tomato sauce

- 100g pitted black olives , roughly chopped

- 1 tbsp capers , drained

- small handful parsley , chopped

Instructions

1. Cook the spaghetti in a large pan of boiling salted water according to pack instructions.

2. Meanwhile, make the sauce.

3. Heat the oil in a medium pan and cook the garlic for 1 min.

4. Add the chilli flakes, tomatoes and sardines, breaking up roughly with a wooden spoon.

5. Heat for 2-3 mins, then stir in the olives, capers and most of the parsley.

6. Mix well to combine.

7. Drain the pasta, reserving a couple of tbsp of the water.

8. Add the pasta to the sauce and mix well, adding the reserved water if the sauce is a little thick.

9. Divide between 4 bowls and sprinkle with the remaining parsley.

Squash & barley salad with balsamic vinaigrette

Preparation time

30 minutes

Ingredients

- 1 butternut squash , peeled and cut into long pieces

- 1 tbsp olive oil

- 250g pearl barley

- 300g Tenderstem broccoli , cut into medium-size pieces

- 100g SunBlush tomato , sliced

- 1 small red onion , diced

- 2 tbsp pumpkin seeds

- 1 tbsp small capers , rinsed

- 15 black olives , pitted

- 20g pack basil , chopped

For the dressing

- 5 tbsp balsamic vinegar

- 6 tbsp extra-virgin olive oil

- 1 tbsp Dijon mustard

- 1 garlic clove , finely chopped

Instructions

1. Heat oven to 200C/fan 180C/gas 6.

2. Place the squash on a baking tray and toss with olive oil.

3. Roast for 20 mins.

4. Meanwhile, boil the barley for about 25 mins in salted water until tender, but al dente.

5. While this is happening, whisk the dressing ingredients in a small bowl, then season with salt and pepper.

6. Drain the barley, then tip it into a bowl and pour over the dressing. Mix well and let it cool.

7. Boil the broccoli in salted water until just tender, then drain and rinse in cold water. Drain and pat dry.

8. Add the broccoli and remaining ingredients to the barley and mix well.

9. This will keep for 3 days in the fridge and is delicious warm or cold.

Chicken Casserole

Preparation time

1 hour 20 minutes

Ingredients

- 2 tbsp sunflower oil

- 400g boneless, skinless chicken thigh , trimmed and cut into chunks

- 1 onion , finely chopped

- 3 carrots , finely chopped

- 3 celery sticks, finely chopped

- 2 thyme sprigs or ½ tsp dried

- 1 bay leaf , fresh or dried

- 600ml vegetable or chicken stock

- 2 x 400g / 14oz cans haricot beans , drained

- chopped parsley , to serve

Instructions

1. Heat the oil in a large pan, add the chicken, then fry until lightly browned.

2. Add the veg, then fry for a few mins more.

3. Stir in the herbs and stock.

4. Bring to the boil.

5. Stir well, reduce the heat, then cover and cook for 40 mins, until the chicken is tender.

6. Stir the beans into the pan, then simmer for 5 mins.

7. Stir in the parsley and serve with crusty bread.

Chargrilled turkey with quinoa tabbouleh & tahini dressing

Preparation time

35 minutes

Ingredients

- 200g quinoa

- ½ cucumber , cut into 1cm chunks

- 175g cherry tomato , halved

- 3 spring onions , finely sliced

- handful parsley , roughly chopped

- handful coriander , roughly chopped

- 1 tbsp olive oil , plus 1 tsp

- juice 1 lemon

- 4 turkey steaks

- For the tahini dressing

- 1½ tbsp tahini paste

- 1½ tbsp low-fat yogurt

- juice ½ lemon

- ½ garlic clove, crushed

- ½ tsp clear honey

Instructions

1. Tip the quinoa into a saucepan and pour over 600ml water.

2. Cover with a lid and bring to the boil.

3. Turn down and simmer until the water has evaporated (just as you'd cook rice) – about 20 mins.

4. Take off the lid and leave to cool while you prepare the turkey and salad.

5. Tip the cucumber, tomatoes, spring onions and herbs into a large mixing bowl.

6. Pour over 1 tbsp olive oil and lemon juice, season well and mix everything together.

7. Heat a griddle pan and, when smoking hot, rub the turkey steaks with 1 tsp olive oil.

8. Cook for about 5 mins on each side, depending on thickness.

9. Stir together all the dressing ingredients along with 3 tbsp water.

10. Toss the quinoa together with the salad and arrange on plates.

11. Cut the turkey into thick slices, pile up on the quinoa and drizzle over the dressing.

Garlic & herb bulgur wheat

Preparation time

20 minutes

Ingredients

- 200g bulgur wheat

- 175g frozen peas

- For the dressing

- 6 tbsp garlic oil

- juice 1 lemon

- handful of herbs , such as (mint, parsley, chives), roughly chopped

Instructions

1. Cook the bulgur wheat in boiling salted water for 15 mins or until tender, adding the peas for the final 3 mins of cooking.

2. Make the dressing by combining the oil, lemon juice and seasoning.

3. Stir the herbs through the drained bulgur wheat and peas with the dressing.

Sweet potato falafels with coleslaw

Preparation time

1 hour 10 minutes

Ingredients

For the falafels

- 1 large or 2 small sweet potatoes , about 700g/1lb 9oz in total
- 1 tsp ground cumin
- 2 garlic cloves , chopped
- 2 tsp ground coriander
- handful coriander leaves , chopped

- juice ½ lemon

- 100g plain or gram flour

- 1 tbsp olive oil

- 4 wholemeal pitta breads

- 4 tbsp reduced-fat hummus

- For the coleslaw

- 2 tbsp red wine vinegar

- 1 tbsp golden caster sugar

- 1 small onion , finely sliced

- 1 medium carrot , grated

- ¼ each white and red cabbage , shredded

Instructions.

1. Heat oven to 200C/180C fan/gas 6.

2. Microwave sweet potato whole for 8-10 mins until tender.

3. Leave to cool a little, then peel.

4. Put the potato, cumin, garlic, ground and fresh coriander, lemon juice and flour into a large bowl.

5. Season, then mash until smooth. Using a tablespoon, shape mix and into 20 balls.

6. Put on an oiled baking sheet, bake for around 15 mins until the bases are golden brown, then flip over and bake for 15 mins more until brown all over.

7. Meanwhile, stir the vinegar and sugar together in a large bowl until the sugar has

dissolved, toss through the onion, carrot and cabbage, then leave to marinate for 15 mins.

8. To serve, toast the pittas, then split. Fill with salad, a dollop of hummus and the falafels.